Kidney Cleansing 101

The Ultimate Guide To Kidney Health And Overall Well-Being

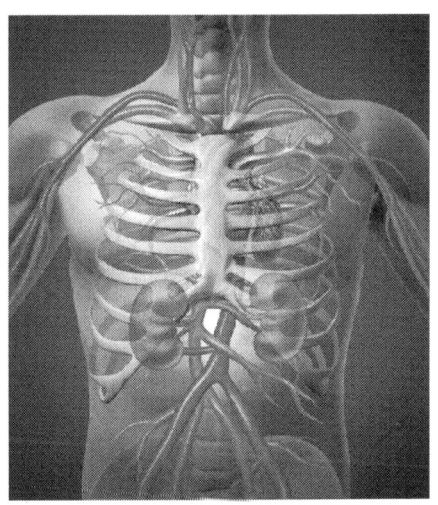

By

Fhilcar Faunillan

Table of Contents

INTRODUCTION

I want to thank you and congratulate you for downloading the book, *"Kidney Cleansing 101: The Ultimate Guide To Kidney Health and Overall Well-being"*.

This book contains proven steps and strategies on how to cleanse your kidney. It also contains recipes that can change your overall well-being.

There have been countless articles on how to clean our kidneys, but in this book, we focus on the importance of our kidneys, the causes of kidney malfunctions and even recipes for kidney detox.

In this book, we will show you different ways to protect yourself from kidney failures, combine kidney-cleaning foods like: watermelon, lemon juice, berries, ginger, turmeric, etc., and make them into delicious meals or drinks, and even get you tips to protecting your kidney.

After reading this book, you will see a significant increase in your energy, mood and your overall well-being.

Thanks again for downloading this book, I hope you enjoy it!

CW01501964

the owned by the owners themselves, not affiliated with this document.

Chapter 1 - The Kidney And Its Functions

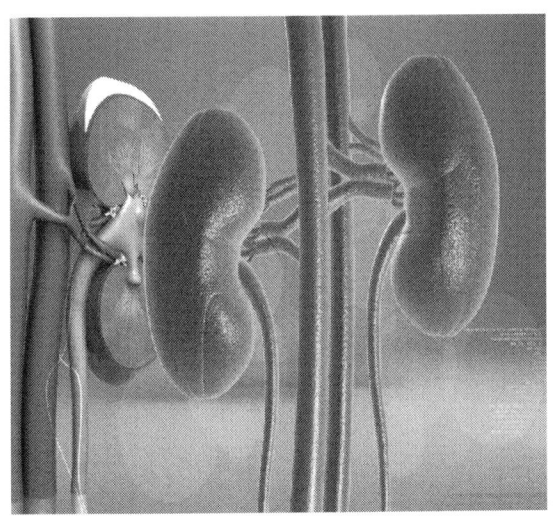

What are these so-called Kidneys?

Kidneys are body organs that are located on either side of our spine, near the lowest level of the rib cage. Each of us are born with two kidneys, both of them having about the size of our fists. And each of these kidneys contain functioning units called nephrons. Each nephron consists of a tiny blood vessel that aids in filtering. This unit is called glomerulus and it is attached to a tubule. Every time blood passes through the glomerulus, the blood is filtered and the remaining fluid passes through the tubule. The residue inside the tubule is then mixed with water or chemicals which is then excreted as urine.

Why are our Kidneys so important?

Although our kidneys may only be as small as our fists, interestingly, they play a huge and important role in our body's overall health and well-being. They perform a number of tasks that keep the body in a state of homeostasis. The kidneys are responsible for the regulation of water, blood pressure, and red blood cells, as well as the production of hormones, and removal of wastes. These functions are done well enough by the kidneys with proper nourishment and care.

Functions of the Kidneys

1. Help in regulating water in the body

In order for our body to work well, we need to have an ample amount of water. This is the reason why 75 percent of our body is made up of water. Water can help us maintain the health of every cell in our body, help our bloodstream flowing, eliminate the excess electrolytes in our body, regulate the temperature of our body through sweating, moisten the mucus in our lungs and mouth, lubricate the joints, reduce the risks of getting cysts by keeping our bladder from bacteria, aid the intestines in digestion and prevent us from getting constipation, moisturize the skin so that it can maintain its appearance and texture, and carry oxygen and nutrients to our cells.

2. Help remove wastes from the body

Our body needs homeostasis — a sense of balance. For our body to function properly, the substances in our blood and our body must be kept at a normal level. It is then the kidney's job to eliminate the excess minerals like sodium and potassium as waste through urination. It also keeps the calcium level normal so that the formation of bones are perfectly done.

3. Produce the necessary hormones

Kidneys also produce hormones that are necessary for the body to function and develop well. These hormones regulate the blood pressure, creation of red blood cells, as well as the return of calcium in the intestine.

4. Regulate blood pressure

In order to filter the blood, the kidneys need to have constant pressure. When there is not enough pressure to let the blood through for filtration, the blood vessels here engage in the process of constriction and retention, making it difficult to maintain the normal blood pressure needed by the body and the kidneys.

Renin, along with another hormone known as angiotensin, are produced by the kidneys in order to help regulate the contraction and expansion of the blood vessels including the amount of sodium and fluid which the body retains.

5. Regulate our red blood cells

Just like our whole system, our kidneys too need oxygen in order to work well. When they do not get enough of it, they tell the brain by sending a call: through the erythroprotein. This is a kind of hormone that signals the bone marrow to release more red blood cells that contain the right amount of oxygen that is needed for the kidneys' processing.

Chapter 2 - Kidney Failure: What Does It Mean to You?

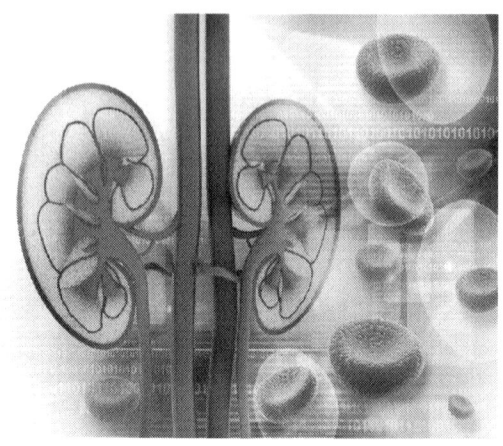

What is Kidney Failure?

Kidney failure occurs when the kidneys lose the ability to filter waste from the blood. There are two kinds of kidney failure, namely:

a) Acute Kidney Failure (AKF); and

b) Chronic Kidney Failure (CKF).

Acute Kidney Failure happens when the kidney suddenly stops and fails to perform its job of filtering the blood off of excess salt, fluids, and other wastes that may, later on, accumulate. AKF develops for a few hours or days, relatively shorter than Chronic Kidney Failure and usually affects those who are hospitalized and receiving intensive care for various reasons.

Chronic Kidney Failure, on the other hand, is the decreased function of the kidney. It is considered a Chronic Kidney Failure when the decreased function of the kidney lasts longer than 4 months. This kind of failure may be dangerous due to its unnoticeable symptoms. The symptoms may not be noticed until it's too late and the kidneys are irreparable. If the kidneys are unable to do their job, the body becomes overloaded with toxins, and that may lead to an unfortunate death.

Causes of Kidney Failure

It is very important to know if the kidney failure has happened suddenly (acute) or over a long period of time (chronic).

For Acute Kidney Failure, the following are the possible causes:

1) Lack of blood flowing in our kidneys

2) A direct hit or severe damage to the kidney

4) Blockage of the urinary track

5) Traumatic injury that involves blood loss

6) Dehydration

7) Obstruction of the flow of urine, just like enlarged prostate

8) Damage to the kidneys caused by drugs and toxins

9) Pregnancy complications

10) Other disorders may also trigger AKF, such as malignant hypertension, scleroderma, and transfusion reaction

For Chronic Kidney Failure, the following are the possible causes:

1) Type 1 or Type 2 Diabetes

2) High Blood pressure

3) Immune system deficiency like HIV/AIDS and Hepatitis B and Hepatitis C

4) Urinary Tract Infection (UTI) within the kidneys (pyelonephritis) which can lead to the scarring of the kidneys after it heals

5) Inflammation in the tiny filters within the kidney (glomeruli)

6) Polycystic kidney disease, wherein cysts filled with fluid form within the kidneys over time (This is the most common cause of Chronic Kidney Failure)

7) Congenital defects, this is present at birth which are usually a result of a malformation that may have affected the kidneys; these defects can usually be found in babies whilst they are in the womb

8) Long term exposure to some drugs and chemicals specifically NSAIDs (nonsteroidal anti-inflammatory drugs)

Symptoms of Kidney Failure

There are a lot of symptoms and signs that would help you identify kidney failure. The following are listed below. If you are experiencing any or a combination of these symptoms, you may want to consult your doctor immediately.

- ➢ Low amount of urine when urinating

- ➢ Swelling of the feet, ankles and legs; usually caused by the failure of the kidneys to remove water wastes that they get stored in these parts instead

- ➢ Shortness of breath for no apparent reason

- ➢ Fatigue or drowsiness

- ➢ Nausea and vomiting

- ➢ Confusion or dull thinking

- ➢ Pain or pressure in the chest

- ➢ Seizures

- ➢ High Blood Pressure

- ➢ Changes in the amount of urine especially at night

- ➢ Changes in the appearance, like color and cloudiness, of the urine

- ➢ Blood mixed in the urine

- ➢ Pain specifically in the kidney area or the sides of the lower back

- ➢ Loss of appetite

- ➢ Difficulty in sleeping and poor quality of sleep

- ➢ Headaches

- ➢ Lack of concentration

- ➢ Itchiness everywhere

- ➢ Metallic taste in the mouth and bad breath

Diagnosis

When you are experiencing most of the said symptoms, you may want to have your kidneys on red alert and engage in different tests to check your kidneys' condition. These are the different ways to diagnose kidney failure:

1) Urinalysis – this is a test that would analyze and evaluate a

sample of your urine. This is used to asses a lot of disorders. Among these are diabetes and Urinary Tract Infection (UTI). Urinalysis involves analyzing the content and the concentration of one's urine. Abnormalities like cloudiness in color or increased levels of protein in the urine are observed through this diagnostic process.

2) Urine Measurements – is yet another test that can measure the amount of urine a person has. The urine measurement is regularly done in order to see if there is a decrease in urine. Having low urine output usually means that there is a blockage in the urinary tract and perhaps a problem in your kidneys' filtration process.

3) Blood Samples – this kind of test usually checks the blood to see if there are any abnormalities in it. If the blood has different substances within it, it usually means that the kidney was unable to filter the blood properly.

4) Imaging – this is a kind of testing that requires an imaging equipment like ultrasound, magnetic resonance imaging (MRI), or computerized tomography (CT) scans. This method of diagnosis can give one a clear image of the kidneys thereby providing ease in determining whether there is a blockage or any kind of physical damage and abnormalities of the said parts.

5) Kidney Tissue Sample – for this test, a kidney biopsy would be needed to get a kidney tissue sample. Biopsies are procedures that are performed while a person is awake wherein a local anesthetic is used to reduce and/or eliminate pain. A biopsy needle is then used so that it can be inserted in the skin all the way to the kidney. X-rays and ultrasounds can be used to assist the physician while he or she is performing this procedure.

Remedies and Treatment

There are various remedies for one who is faced with kidney failure. However, you should take note that once you have started with any of these methods and later on you feel like shifting to another kind of treatment, always ask your doctor first before trying something else. Most of the time, you would also need two or more treatments in order to fully cure kidney failure. Take for example, if you decide to have a kidney transplant, you would still need to undergo a series of dialysis in order to make the kidney useable.

The remedies available include the following:

1) Dialysis – this is a treatment wherein a machine is used to act as kidneys. Dialysis does not completely cure kidney failure, but it does extend your life.

2) Kidney Transplant – this is an operation that replaces your current kidney with a healthy one. The kidney may come from a

donor or a diseased person. The only downside to this is that you would have to wait a long time to be able to get a donor for kidney transplant. Usually, this new kidney would work immediately, but there are also some factors that need to be checked in order to see if the kidney is compatible with the patient. If rejection happens, dialysis is needed immediately and a second transplant can happen.

3) Hemodialysis – this is a treatment that would remove wastes and fluids from the blood. During this procedure, the blood is pumped through soft tubes into a dialysis machine where the blood goes inside a *dialyzer*. After the blood is filtered, it is then sent back to your blood stream. This is usually done for 3-5 hours, 3 times a week. However, if this is performed on a daily basis, it can bc done for 1 ½ hours to 2 hours.

4) Peritoneal Dialysis (PD) – this type of dialysis is a home-based treatment which can even be done

while you are sleeping. This procedure must be done daily to ensure efficiency. You will need a catheter (a flexible tube that is inserted through a narrow opening in your body) inside the abdomen. Unlike hemodialysis, this procedure cleans your blood while it is inside your body. With this procedure, the lining of the abdomen (peritoneum) acts like a natural filter than can clean the blood.

How can you stop the symptoms of Chronic Kidney Failure from getting worse?

Here are different ways to keep your kidney failure from getting worse:

> ➤ Controlling the current health problems that you may have

> ➤ Treating minor/early complications of kidney failure

- Preventing or managing heart diseases

- Taking in medications like angiotensin converting enzymes (ACEs) or angiotensin receptor blockers (ARBs); it has been proven that these medications can help protect the kidney's ability to function

- Losing weight if needed

- Cutting down on your salt intake in order to control blood pressure

- If you are a diabetic, monitoring the blood sugar and following all or any prescribed diet and/or medication is highly recommended

- Treating heart and blood vessel problems

- Seeking cure for anemia (when the blood cell count is low)

- Treating any bone and mineral problems

- Addressing poor nutritional health

Chapter 3 - Kidney Stones: Symptoms, Causes, and Cure

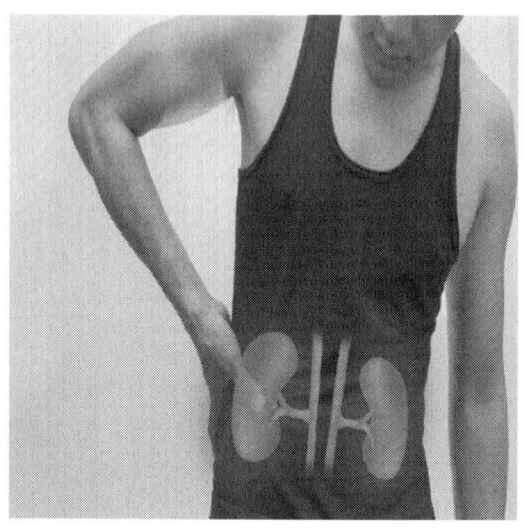

What are Kidney Stones?

Kidney stones are stones that are found within the kidney, in the ureter (the tube that drains urine from the kidney), or in the bladder. The medical term for these stones is Nephrolithiasis. While our kidneys are filtering our blood, the kidneys create urine. Sometimes, the mineral wastes from our blood may stick together and can therefore turn into stones. These stones are usually made up of calcium oxalate, which are the result of having an accumulated dissolved minerals in the inner lining of our kidney. These stones can even grow up to the size of a single golf ball and can even have a sharp and crystal structure. Sometimes, these stones can even be too large that it can be stuck in the ureter and even cause enlargement of the tube.

Having kidney stones in the body can manifest a lot of side effects. Some stones can be so small that no pain can be felt when urinating or it can be big enough to cause extreme pain every time a person excretes urine.

Prevalence of Kidney Stones

Studies show that 1 out 10 Americans, at one point in their lives, will be suffering from kidney stone. And every year, at least half a million people are rushed to the hospitals because of this kidney problem. Most of the time, this affects White Americans who are males.

Kinds of Kidney Stones

1) Calcium stones – most of the kidney stones are calcium stones. They are in a form of calcium oxalate. These oxalates are substances that are normally found in our everyday food. Some of these foods, like nuts and chocolate, contain more oxalate levels than the usual. Moreover, having high doses of vitamin D, intestinal bypass surgery and other metabolic disorders may likewise increase the concentration of calcium oxalate in the urine.

2) Struvite stones – these stones come as a reaction to infections such as Urinary Tract Infection or UTI. They can increase rapidly in size without warning.

3) Uric acid stones – these stones normally form when people do not drink enough fluids or those who lose fluids rapidly. This is usually common to individuals who are on a high-protein diet or those who have gout. Some genetic factors can also increase the chances of having uric acid stones.

4) Cystine stones – These stones form in people who excrete too much amino acids. This is usually a hereditary disorder.

Symptoms of Kidney Stones

A kidney stone may not show symptoms when it's too small. The symptoms usually involve pain in the kidney, ureter or bladder area. There may be a sudden and severe pain that may get worse in waves. People often describe this pain as the worst pain that they have experienced in their entire lives. However this pain may vary depending on the position in the urinary tract as it can move whenever someone urinates and the stone may change places depending on the intensity of the urine.

Here are the symptoms of kidney stones:

1) Pain in the kidney (a stone that may have been stuck in the kidney can cause this)

2) Renal colic (this is a severe pain which may go away and come back and can also be constant. This is because of a stone that is stuck in the ureter. Pain is caused during urination.)

3) Blood in urine (can be caused by a stone rubbing in the ureter, color may vary, it can be pink, red or brown)

4) Infection (usually results to having a fever)

5) Severe pain in the side and back (this is usually below the ribs)

6) Pain that can spread to the lower abdomen and the groin

7) Pain during urination

8) Foul-smelling urine

9) Cloudy urine

10) Nausea and vomiting

11) Constant need to urinate

12) Peeing more than usual

13) Urinating small amounts of urine

14) Feeling of restlessness and the inability to lie still

When should you see a doctor?

Normally, a person should see a doctor regularly to ensure good health. This may be a problem for people who are busy or just afraid to go to the doctor.

Here are conditions as to when you should see a doctor:

1) When you have pain that's so severe that you can't sit still or lie down still or even find a comfortable position;

2) When the pain can also make you nauseated or even cause you to vomit;

3) When the pain is accompanied by fever and/or chills;

4) When there is blood found in your urine;

5) When you have difficulty in passing urine; or

6) When you are having waves and waves of sharp pain in your back, abdomen, or side.

Possible causes

There may be no single cause for these stones, but one thing is sure, dehydration is the common cause for all of them.

Other causes may be:

1) Consuming a high-protein, low fiber diet;

2) Inactivity or being bed-bound;

3) Kidney stones run in the family;

4) Having several urinary tract infections or kidney infections;

5) Having a kidney stone before, usually before you were 25 years old;

6) Only 1 of your kidneys are functional;

7) You have undergone intestinal bypass or if you have a disease on your small intestine; or

8) A buildup of any of the following: calcium, ammonia, uric acid and cysteine (an amino acid that helps with the building of protein)

Treatment

Kidney stones may still be manageable and curable. Here are ways to cure and/treat kidney stones:

1) Using sound waves in order to break kidney stones (these strong shockwaves can destroy large stones);

2) Surgery to remove large stones inside the kidney;

3) Using a ureteroscope (a thin tube with a camera attached) that is passed through the urethra to the bladder to the ureter;

4) Undergoing a parathyroid gland surgery;

5) Using pain medicine (for small stones or stones that are not that dangerous);

6) Drinking enough or more fluids; or

7) Lifestyle changes for better health habits.

Chapter 4 - Kidney Diseases and their Prevalence

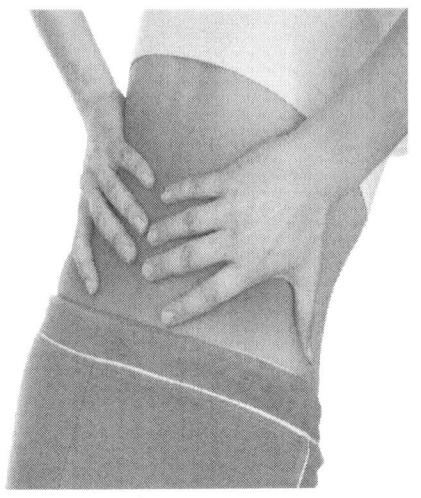

Prevalence of Kidney Problems in United States of America

Studies show that 1 out of 3 American adults are at risk for having any kidney disease and 26 million of them already have kidney problems. The fact remains though that despite the alarming number, there are still a lot of people who have been unchecked for kidney problems. For that reason, extra care and awareness should be spread about the possible complications most especially that diseases involving the kidneys land on the 9th spot on being the leading cause of death in the United States, killing a significant number of people even higher compared to that of prostate and breast cancer. And just in 2013, kidney disease killed more than 47, 000 people in USA and every single day, 12 people die waiting for a healthier kidney transplant.

These facts and figures have not been presented to scare you off but make you think that your kidneys should not be taken for granted. As early as possible, engage in activities and lifestyle choices that would be better for them.

Chronic Kidney Disease

This is a kidney problem that involves the continuous and long-term loss of the ability of the kidneys to do their job. Worse comes to worst, this may even lead to the building up of wastes in the body that can cause further danger like kidney failure.

Chronic Kidney Disease is often linked with other diseases such as high blood pressure, diabetes, nerve problems, and anemia with diabetes and high blood pressure and are identified as its main causes. Concentrated blood sugar can cause damage to many other organs in the body and that includes the kidneys and blood vessels in it. High blood pressure, on the other hand, can cause damage to the walls of the blood vessels as its lack of control can damage the blood vessels as well. These blood vessels are necessary in passing through the kidneys for excess waste removal. If these vessels are damaged, the process of filtration of the kidneys will also be affected negatively.

Acute Kidney Injury

Acute Kidney Injury is common among older patients in hospitals. This happens when the kidneys cannot sieve the toxins from your blood. This is when the function of filtration slows down and results to the inability to keep body fluid, electrolytes, and acid-base balance in the body.

The common symptoms of acute kidney injury include nausea, vomiting, confusion, dehydration, rashes, and bruises. This may develop fast even just a few hours or days. However, as it is acute, it can still be reversed with proper treatment.

Kidney Cysts

There are two types of kidney cysts that may develop. One is majorly affected by genetic make-up and the other is acquired.

Polycystic kidney disease, which is most often passed on among family members, take and develop the cysts on normal tissues, which can be the kidneys. The kidneys may swell and enlarge, causing them function poorly or not function at all anymore. In worst cases, the cysts may completely damage the kidneys and this can lead to kidney failure. This is often observed with the smearing pain at the sides of the lower back, headaches, blood in the urine, and even the development of urinary tract infection.

On the other hand, Acquired Cystic Kidney Disease often affects those who have undergone or are still undergoing dialysis, despite the lack of this in the genetic line. In this kidney problem, the kidneys are not enlarged or swelled. This often has no evident symptoms and most often, the cysts formed in this condition are not really very harmful.

Kidney Cancer

The kidney cancer forms along the linings of the tubes inside your kidneys that cleanse and filter the blood off of wastes. This can be very prone to those who engage in excessive smoking, drinking of pain relievers for a long time, and under the genetic lines of the family. This becomes more and more possible for these people to acquire this kidney problem as they age.

The known symptoms of kidney cancer include the presence of blood in the urine, lump in the abdominal area, loss of appetite and weight for no apparent reason (even without dieting or exercising), and pain in the lower sides of the back part of the body where the kidneys are nearly located.

The treatment of kidney cancer depends on many factors: your age, overall health, and the status of the cancer itself. The possible treatments may include the usual surgery, chemotherapy, and radiation. Biologic is also a tentative treatment as it can improve the body's ability to fight off the cancer cells. Targeted therapy is another possible treatment that involves the production of substances that would attack the cancer cells only and not include the normal cells.

Urinary Tract Infection

Urinary Tract Infection is an endocrine system problem that does not only involve the kidneys but the other parts of the system as well like the ureters, bladder, and urethra. This infection in the urinary system is the second most common infection in the body and can affect any age and sex but is mostly common among women.

The symptoms of UTI include pain when urinating, fever, fatigue, urge to pee every so often even without drinking lots of water, lower belly pressure and discomfort, pain in the sides of the lower back near the kidneys, and the reddening, dulling, and stinking of urine produced.

For treatment, you may consult your doctor. This problem can still be treated by antibiotics depending on the prescription of the doctor.

Chapter 5 - Natural Kidney Cleansers

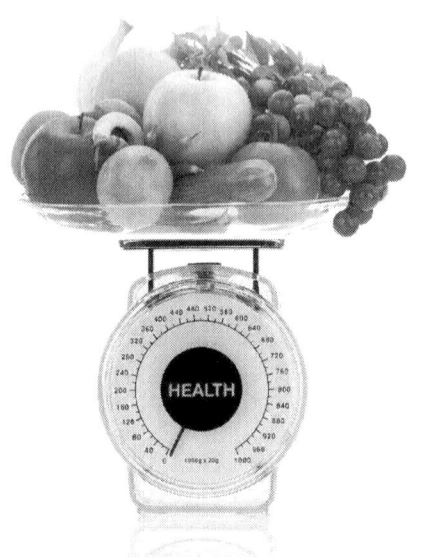

The usual and known treatments for different kidney problems are undeniably quite expensive and may even give you some side effects. However, there are alternative cures and preventive ways of dealing with these problems that are way cheaper and easier to access, especially when some of these alternatives can be found in your garden or kitchen at home. The following are examples of organic fruits, vegetables, and herbs that are natural sources for kidney care:

Grapes

Grapes are rich in antioxidants and nutrients that can facilitate better detoxification in the body and thus helping out the kidneys in flushing out the excess wastes. Make grapes as part of your diet. Munch on these freshly-washed fruits.

Cranberries

Cranberries contain quinine that is then transformed into hippuric acid. This transformed compound is then used by the body in cleaning the kidneys and urinary tract off of urea and other bacteria.

Onions

Onions, along with kidney beans, peas, and soybeans, are rich in arginine. This is an essential amino acid that helps the kidneys get rid of ammonia. The onions may be boiled and then blended with the water from which it was boiled. Simply mix it well in a blender.

Garlic

Garlic is a great cleansing agent too which if consumed, may help in increasing urine production as well as the flushing out of the urine from the kidneys.

Cucumber and Sprouts

These are also organic sources of kidney cleansers that can improve the production of urine as they contain high fluids that can flush the kidney and even bladder stones out.

Ginger

Ginger contain high levels of antioxidant compounds that facilitate blood purification and the kidney's filtration of the wastes in the body.

Turmeric

Turmeric is good for kidney inflammation and infection as they contain anti-inflammatory compounds.

Parsley

Parsley is good for cleansing the kidneys as it helps in flushing out the excess wastes. This is best for kidney stones and urinary tract infection. This may be added as garnish in your food, as salad, or even as tea.

Red Clover

This is another diuretic, or a kidney cleanser that facilitates the flushing of toxins by increasing the urine production of the person who consumes it.

Dandelion

All parts of a dandelion can be dried or used fresh and can be brewed into tea. This dandelion tea is best for improving kidney cleansing, water retention, urine production, and strengthening of the kidneys.

Nettle

Nettle is an herb that helps in keeping the water flow through the bladder and the kidneys in order to flush the bacteria and other wastes away. It is also rich in iron that can facilitate in blood building. This can be dried or used fresh for tea brewing. Just soak it in hot water for 10 to 15 minutes, let it cool down a bit, and then drink immediately to experience its detoxifying effect.

Cabbage

Cabbages are rich in many vitamins and minerals that are good for the body. They have high phytochemical content which aids in the fighting off of free radicals, Vitamin C, Vitamin B6, folic acid, and fiber. More so, cabbage contains a very little amount of potassium which makes it safer for the kidneys.

These are easy to include in different recipes. You can have them as coleslaw or toppings. And you can have cabbages steamed, boiled, or even baked.

Cauliflower

Cauliflowers are super foods for our kidneys since they contain not only fiber but Vitamin C and folate as well. More so, they also help in neutralizing toxic substances, as they work hand in hand with the processes done by the liver.

You can serve cauliflowers as you prefer. They can either be steamed, boiled, or mashed, and mixed with different recipes.

Raspberries

Aside from Vitamin C, manganese, fiber, folate, and Vitamin B, raspberries are also rich in ellagic acid which aids in the neutralizing of free radicals in the body. Additionally, raspberries also contain antioxidants called anthocyanins. They are good for preventing cancer cells and tumor growth, and may help you avoid having kidney cancer or even any other cancer.

You can top raspberries on your breakfast oats or even have it fresh as a side serving.

Strawberries

Like raspberries, strawberries also contain high levels of Vitamin C, fiber, and manganese. Aside from those, they also contain anti-cancer and anti-inflammatory properties that help in preventing damage to your organs, including your kidneys.

You can include strawberries in your breakfast oats, have them as a side serving, juice them up, or blend them as a smoothie.

Cherries

Cherries have antioxidants and phytochemicals in them. These substances are good for the heart and while they are good for the heart, they support the kidneys in order for it to function well. They can reduce inflammation developments in the system.

Cherries can be served as snacks, toppings, or even as sauce to lamb or pork slices.

Egg Whites

Eggs may be high in protein, which when consumed highly will result to a kidney problem. But more so, out of all the protein sources, only egg whites have the lowest amount of phosphorous.

You can have these egg whites served as omelets or as fillings for sandwiches, depending on your desired recipe.

Fish

Fish is a lean protein source that, if consumed in significant amounts, will put the kidneys in danger. Which is why, fish is only recommended in your meal plan at least twice a week. Aside from being a good source of protein necessary for your body's building, fish is also rich in omega-3, a good anti-inflammatory fat that helps fight cancer cells and heart disease by lowering the bad cholesterol in the system and in turn raising the good cholesterol.

Salmon, Albacore Tuna, Herring, Mackerel, and Rainbow trout are some of the fishes with high omega-3 content.

Chapter 6 - Basic Kidney Cleanse Diet

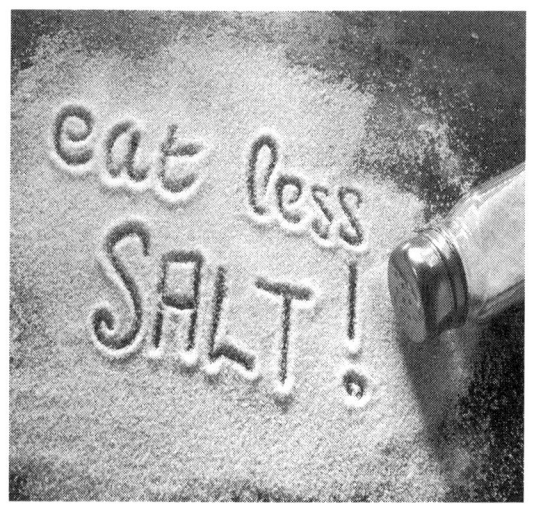

What you eat and drink may either worsen or improve your kidney condition. Some foods are better for your kidneys' functioning as compared to other foods and you will need their nutrients in your diet. Eating right is a way of keeping your kidneys in good, if not better, health.

You do not have to give up all of these foods entirely. You just have to take them in modicum amounts that will be enough to nourish your body without stressing out your kidneys. How do you do that?

1. Select foods with lower sodium and salt content

Your body only needs less than 2,300 milligrams of sodium. Excess sodium will have to be released from the body as waste in any form. Lesser salt and sodium in the system will help in balancing the blood pressure.

So when you select foods, watch out for their sodium content. Check the labels and as much as possible, cut off on consuming processed foods. They contain high amounts of sodium in them as these help in keeping the food in their preserved state. If you decide to buy processed food, at least, rinse these canned vegetables, fruits, meat, beans, and fish with water.

However, it would be a whole safer and cheaper to opt for fresher fruits and vegetables and invest on spices to give flavor to your food rather than adding too much preservatives and salt. You may use sodium-free seasonings and herbs to add up to the food that you would cook.

2. Consume the right proteins in just the right amounts

Protein is needed by the body especially for building muscles. However, a with high-protein diet, adverse effects may happen to your kidneys' functioning. Protein fills you up because it stays longer in your stomach as it needs a lot of energy to get digested. This long processing stresses out the kidneys and causes it to *hyper filtrate* instead — a state of increased pressure for the kidneys to filtrate wastes. In the long run, constant hyper filtration of the kidneys may cause them damage, which is why you have to be careful with your protein intake as well.

You do not have to give up protein entirely as it is one of the basic nutrients needed by the body, the key here is to consume it in the right amounts from healthy protein sources.

You may opt for animal-protein foods such as chicken, meat, eggs, dairy, and fish. Or, you may consume plan-protein foods like beans, nuts, and grains. Consider talking to your dietician for specifications of protein combination especially if you have a kidney problem.

3. Choose what is healthy for your heart

Avoid fatty foods since they store up in your blood vessels, heart, and kidneys, causing these parts to function poorly in the long run. Instead of deep frying your food, you may choose to grill, broil, roast, stir-fry, or bake them. Or if you cannot give up frying entirely, you may use a non-stick cooking spray or a little amount of olive oil.

When you prepare your meat, like pork or beef, trim the fat off by cutting it away. For chicken meat, remove the skin as it is where most of the cholesterol are stored.

Foods that are healthy for your heart include lean meat like loin or round, fish, beans, vegetables, fruits, and low-fat dairy such as milk, yogurt, and cheese.

4. Cut back on phosphorous

When your kidneys are not in a healthy and normal state, you may want to cut back on consuming foods with high content of phosphorus. Phosphorus is a mineral needed for building strong bones. However, our bodies only need a certain amount of it. The kidneys regulate this to a balance by flushing off excess phosphorus out of the body. If the kidneys fail to do so or do this poorly, phosphorus will accumulate in the blood and will decrease the amount of calcium in it. With decreased calcium content in the blood, you may be prone to developing bone diseases.

You may want to check the labels of the packed foods that you consume. Look for phosphorus or PHOS content on ingredient labels. There may also be added phosphorus even on deli and fresh meat and poultry so may want to ask the butcher to help you choose those without added amounts of phosphorus.

Foods high in phosphorus include meat, egg, chicken, fish, bran cereals and oats, dairy, bean, lentils, and nuts. And foods that you may consume instead if you need to cut back on phosphorus intake are fresh fruits and vegetables, corn and rice cereals, bread, pasta, and rice.

5. Give your body the right amount of potassium

Potassium is an essential nutrient for the cells to function well. However, our body needs just the right amount of it. Our kidneys do the regulation of the amount of potassium in the body as it helps in removing the extra potassium through filtration. If the kidneys' functioning is poor, potassium may be stored in the blood. This potassium build-up may lead to further diseases like Addison's disease, muscle and cell damage especially when one is undergoing medication, surgery, or chemotherapy, haemolytic anemia which is a condition that causes the bursting of blood vessels, internal bleeding in the stomach or intestines, and even tumor developments.

To help your nerves, muscles, and kidneys function well, choose foods that have the sufficient amount of potassium needed by your body.

Foods high in potassium include bananas, oranges, potatoes, tomatoes, brown rice, bran cereals and oats, whole wheat bread, whole wheat pasta, beans, and nuts. Foods with low potassium content include apples, peaches, carrots, green beans, white bread, pasta, white rice, and grits.

If you decide to consume canned vegetables and fruits, rinse them first with water before using.

Chapter 7 - Kidney Detoxification

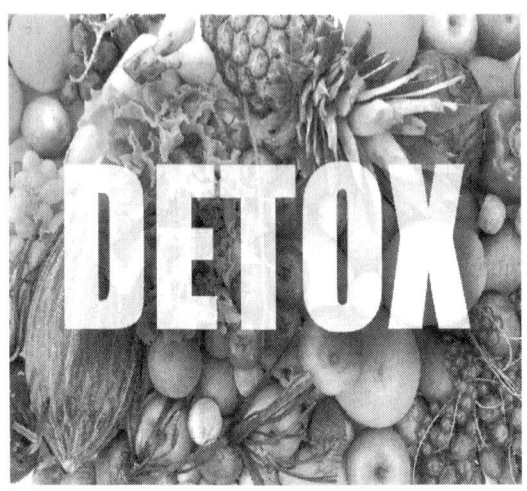

When to Detoxify Your Kidneys

Our kidneys are always at work and giving them utmost care would only be fair to all the hard work they do to keep our body healthy by getting rid of the toxins we take in through what we put in our mouths. When you feel like your body is experiencing some kind of imbalance or so much tiredness that not even sleep or rest can cure then you may consider a kidney cleanse. This is most especially true when you know you have not been feeding your body well for the past few days.

Some people may justify that our body does not really need the process of detoxification since we are equipped with organs that do that job naturally. But with today's extreme exposure to different toxins from what we eat, what we drink, what we apply to our bodies' external parts, and what we environmentally expose ourselves with, we are accumulating more and more toxins that even our body filters could not handle. If we put too much pressure on their functions of cleansing all by themselves, pushing them even to the limits, they may soon crash. So, why wait for this to happen when you know you can do something more about cleansing your own body off of wastes? Give yourself the white flag of detoxification when you start to experience the following:

• When you feel fatigued and stressed out more than you usually feel

- When you are experiencing frequent signs of urinary problems like difficulty in peeing
- When you have had experiences of having kidney stones
- When you feel extra moody than usual due to hormonal imbalance
- When you are having skin problems like rashes, eczema, or acne
- When you get bloated so easily
- When you feel pain after consuming foods high in sodium and preservatives
- When you have poor physical growth and development
- When you have dull and easy to break nails
- When you have terrible balance
- When you have an unexplainable fear
- When you have low sex drive or signs of infertility
- When you experience food intolerances

Benefits of Kidney Detoxification

All the toxins that we consume and excess wastes that our body needs to remove from itself, passes right through the kidneys through the blood stream and its filtration. When too much toxins are taken in and increased amounts of excess wastes may be needed to flush off the system, the kidneys may not be able to function well enough anymore. Thus, they may do their job poorly or not at all. However, with natural detoxification recipes, herbs, and juices, the following benefits for the kidneys and the body may be experienced.

• May dissolve kidney stones and lessen complications

• Flushing out of toxins from the body will reflect clearer and healthier skin

• More physical and mental energy

• Increased hemoglobin content in the blood

• Better quality of sleep

• Relief of lower back pain and other body pains

• Better urinary function and improved urine flow

• Relieve other kidney problem symptoms

Chapter 8 - Kidney Detox Recipes

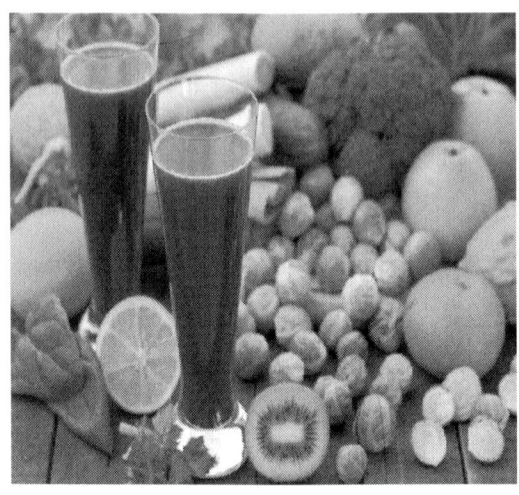

To detox basically means to get rid of the body's toxins. While you may think of drinking that liquid that may be prescribed by your doctor or probably have an over-the-counter liquid drink that would result in constant toilet trips, kidney cleansing need not be an expensive treatment thought as you can make your own detox recipes out of ingredients may be reached easily from your kitchen counters, found in your garden, or even highly available at your grocery stores nearby.

Here are a few recipes that you can make at home in order to cleanse your kidneys:

WATERLEMON JUICE

Yield: 1-2 servings
Preparation time: 10-15 minutes

Ingredients:
4 cups of watermelon
1 peeled lemon

Preparation:
Simply mix all ingredients in a juicer. You can drink it immediately or have it chilled.

ULTIMATE PARSLEY-C JUICE

Yield: 1-2 servings
Preparation time: 10-15 minutes

Ingredients:
½ cup of parsley
2 ribs of celery
1 piece of carrot
1 piece of cucumber

Preparation:
Juice all ingredients and combine together. This is best consumed when chilled.

DANDY APPLES

Yield: 1-2 servings
Preparation time: 10-15 minutes

Ingredients:
3 pieces of dandelion leaves
½ green apple
2 stalks of celery
½ lemon
A chunk of broccoli stalk

Preparation:
Juice all ingredients and combine together.
This is best consumed when chilled.

PURPLE POWER JUICE

Yield: 1-2 servings
Preparation time: 10-15 minutes

Ingredients:
1 cup of radish
1 cup of purple radish
1 rib of celery

Preparation:
Juice all ingredients and combine together.
This is best consumed when chilled.

RAVISHING RADISH

Yield: 1-2 servings
Preparation time: 10-15 minutes

Ingredients:
2 cups of chopped radish
1 rib of celery
1 cucumber
½ lemon

Preparation:
Juice all ingredients and combine together.
This is best consumed when chilled.

DEEP GREEN DETOX

Yield: 1-2 servings
Preparation time: 10-15 minutes

Ingredients:
A handful of spinach
A handful of kale
½ green apple
½ lemon
1 inch piece of ginger
½ cup of fresh parsley

Preparation:
Juice all ingredients and combine together.
This is best consumed when chilled.

DEAD RED DETOX

Yield: 1-2 servings
Preparation time: 10-15 minutes

Ingredients:
½ head of red cabbage
½ lemon
1 piece of cucumber
A chunk of broccoli stalk
¼ cup of fresh cilantro

Preparation:
Juice all ingredients and combine together.
This is best consumed when chilled.

SUMMER ESCAPE

Yield: 1-2 servings
Preparation time: 10-15 minutes

Ingredients:
3 tbsp. of chopped basil
1.5 cups of blueberries
2 pinches of cayenne pepper
½ lime
5 cups of diced watermelon

Preparation:
Juice all ingredients and combine together.
This is best consumed when chilled.

SIMPLY SWEET

Yield: 1-2 servings
Preparation time: 10-15 minutes

Ingredients:
½ lemon
1 large tomato
5 cups of diced watermelon

Preparation:
Juice all ingredients and combine together.
This is best consumed when chilled.

KINKY PINKY DETOX

Yield: 1-2 servings
Preparation time: 10-15 minutes

Ingredients:
1 medium apple
1 orange
1 whole strawberry
1 cup of diced watermelon

Preparation:
Juice all ingredients and combine together.
This is best consumed when chilled.

THE LEMON GRASS DETOX

Yield: 3-5 servings
Preparation 10-15 minutes

Ingredients:
2 cups lemon grass
organic honey
5 cups water for boiling

Procedure:
1. In a pot, add water and bring to boil.
2. Add in lemon grass and bring to boil for 10 minutes.
3. You can drink this as you would your tea and add some honey if desired.

SPARKLY BERRIES

Yield: 1-2 servings
Preparation time: 10-15 minutes

Ingredients:
6 cups of cranberry juice
1 and ½ cups of orange juice
3 cups of ginger ale
Ice cubes

Preparation:
Stir in all ingredients in a pitcher and serve.

BERRY RELAXING

Yield: 1-2 servings
Preparation time: 10-15 minutes

Ingredients:
¾ to 1 cup of ice cubes
3 ounces of cranberry juice
2 ounces of white grapefruit juice

Preparation:
Mix all ingredients in a pitcher and serve.

DETOX WATER

Yield: 5 servings
Preparation: 10 minutes

Ingredients:
¾ pitcher of water
1 lemon or lime, sliced
½ cup parsley
2 tablespoons mint leaves

Preparation:
1. Combine all ingredients together and chill.
2. You can use that as your water for the day.

THE GREEN LIFE DETOX

Yield: 1-2 servings
Preparation time: 5-10 minutes

Ingredients:
2 Granny Smith apples, cored and sliced
½ cup romaine lettuce, chopped
½ cup cilantro
½ cup asparagus

Procedure:
In a high powered blender, combine all ingredients together. Transfer into glass. Chill and consume immediately.

HAWAIIAN CRANNIES

Yield: 1-2 servings
Preparation time: 10-15 minutes

Ingredients:
1 cup of cranberry juice
1 cup of pineapple juice
¼ teaspoon of almond extract
1 to ¼ cups of chilled ginger ale

Preparation:
Combine all ingredients together. This is best consumed when chilled.

FABBERRY

Yield: 1-2 servings
Preparation time: 10-15 minutes

Ingredients:
8 cups of chilled cranberry juice
10 ounces of thawed and pureed frozen
sweetened sliced strawberries
1 teaspoon of vanilla extract
4 cups of chilled ginger ale

Preparation:
Combine together in a smoothie maker.
Transfer to glass and consume immediately.

Chapter 9 - How to Maintain Your Kidneys

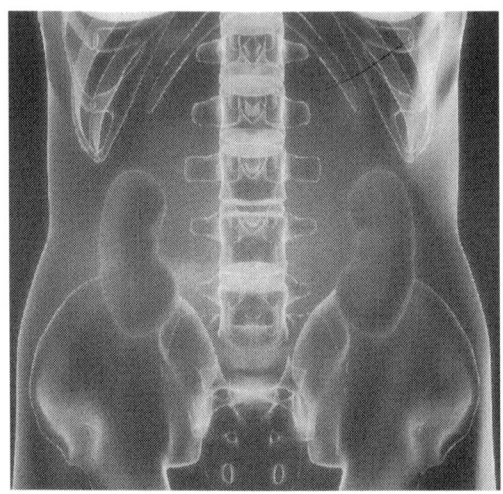

Here are tips on how to maintain and keep your kidneys healthy and to ensure a healthier overall well being:

1. Keep yourself hydrated but do not overdo

Drinking at least 8 glasses of water to keep your body going is not a cliché nor is it a myth. Dehydration is a major cause of developing kidney stones. So drink plenty but enough fluids to keep your kidneys in proper functioning.

Most especially, drink plenty of water when you are under the heat of the sun or strenuous exercise to replenish the fluid you have lost by sweating.

2. Control your glucose level

Many other diseases, like diabetes, are linked with kidney problems. Increased glucose level in the blood, like in Type 2 diabetes puts extra pressure on the kidney's function of filtering excess glucose.

3. Keep a normal blood pressure

Increased blood pressure may thicken the walls of the blood vessels and may also affect the filtration of the kidneys of the blood. Monitor your blood pressure and keep in normal state to avoid complications.

4. Decrease your salt intake

Studies have shown that increased salt intake causes the increased levels of protein in the blood stream. This is a major risk factor in the deterioration of the kidneys' functioning.

5. Opt for healthier foods

By healthier, this means, you should choose fresh fruits and vegetables and lean meat. Make sure you get a balanced diet and not an extreme excess of any mineral as this will put great pressure on the kidneys to filter.

6. Cut back on your alcohol intake

Alcohol may also contain other nutrients like carbohydrates necessary for the body, but in excessive amount what you take in is a bunch of toxins that the kidneys would have to remove from the blood. This direct consumption of toxins may lead to the kidneys to exert double time in its function to get rid of waste.

7. Shed off some weight of needed

Being overweight and obese may be more of a risk factor in adding pressure to your kidneys' work. These may cause you to have increased blood pressure, which is another problem for your kidneys.

8. Engage in physical activities

In order to lose weight and maintain a normal blood pressure, you may engage in regular exercise. Physical activities will also provide you with another outlet to release your toxins, other than just urinating. This way, you may also remove toxins from your body through sweating them off. So what are you waiting for, whether you do your simple household chores, walk your dog around the neighborhood or park, jog or do simple errands, as long as you sweat yourself out, you are doing your kidneys a great favor of helping its job in releasing the toxins out of your body.

9. Quit smoking

It is of common knowledge that smoking whether cigars, cigarettes or any nicotine containing puffs is dangerous to your and everybody's health – either as a first hand or second hand smoker. Smoking also adds up on the accumulated toxins in the body that the kidneys may have to get rid of. With all the other toxins that need to be released, the kidneys will have to exert more effort instead. In the long run, smoking will not only damage your lungs but also impair the kidneys from functioning well or at all.

10. Lessen your caffeine intake

Increased caffeine intake is one of the root cause of developing at type of kidney stone called the calcium oxalate kidney stone. Caffeine puts your natural bodily processes to a halt and even causes one to put on more weight. Excessive accumulation of fats takes a toll on our kidneys.

11. Be careful in taking supplements and other herbal remedies

A wide variety of dietary supplements and other herbal remedies may have different effects on the kidneys but there are those that can severely cause injury. The best way to keep your kidneys safe when you take in these products is to take the advice from your doctor on what is best for you to use, considering the ingredients of these substances.

12. Do not resist your urge to urinate

Holding on your urine for a long time may cause bacteria to grow and dwell in your bladder. This may cause infections and other problems in your urinary system.

So whenever you feel the urge to pee, go and heed to the nearest toilet and relieve yourself. Whenever you are in a middle of an urgent meeting, excuse yourself. There's nothing more important than your kidney's health.

13. Have a Blood and Urine Test

Some kidney problems do not really have obvious signs in their early development. The only best way to know if your kidneys are still functioning well is to have yourself tested. If you have diabetes, high blood pressure, heart disease, family history of kidney problems, obese, African, Asian, or of Aboriginal origin, then you are of increased risk in developing kidney problems. Get yourself tested immediately.

14. Watch your drug medication

Non-steroidal anti-inflammatory drugs like ibuprofen and naproxen, as well as other pain relievers may cause harm to your kidneys. Your kidneys are safe, though, if you only take these drug medications during emergencies or circumstances when the pain can no longer be tolerated. But if these drugs are taken regularly under dependency even in tolerable cases of pain and of high dosages, chances are your kidneys will crash and function poorly instead. Ask your doctor on how you could deal with pain without depending on these drugs for these may only create further damage to your kidneys.

15. Say Goodbye to Soda Consumption

Soft drinks would be very hard on your kidneys. Sodas contain too much sugar and caffeine. These excess wastes will have to be filtered by your kidneys, adding extra pressure on them. In very excessive amounts, these wastes are then formed into stones.

16. Get enough sleep

Sleep is the answer to everything – cell renewal, energy recharge, name it! You need sleep to keep your kidneys in a healthy state. Sleep disruption may also disturb your kidney tissues renewal causing them to get damaged in the long run. So do not overexert yourself all the time, if you need to sleep, then do not deprive yourself. Your kidneys also need it.

17. Watch your protein intake

Protein is good for building your muscles but too much protein in the body also means that there would be an increase in ammonia, protein's by-product which is a toxin that the kidneys will have to neutralize. With too much ammonia in the system, the kidneys will have to double their pressure and effort in working. This may cause them to falter in the long run.

18. Find quick and proper treatment for common infections

Some people have the tendency to shrug off certain infections, especially when they do not really hurt so much. But do not abuse yourself by pushing it off of the limits, coming to the brink of utter exhaustion. Your reluctance of rest and proper healing will also damage your kidneys.

19. Avoid Genetically Modified Foods

Most of the fruits and vegetables that look appallingly pretty, smooth, bigger than the usual size, and flawless are genetically modified. This modification is done for increasing these fruits and vegetables' pest resistance, immunity to herbicides, and increasing crop yields.

But these flawlessly-looking fruits and vegetables actually have ugly effects on our filtering systems in the body. GMOs have high toxicity that would have to be handled by our kidneys and liver. Over the long period of time, this could cause serious damage to these parts.

Instead, opt for organically grown fruits and vegetables. If you also want, you can also grow your own fruits and vegetables so you can make sure that no mutations were done.

20. Say farewell to Dairy Products

Consuming dairy products will translate to an increase of calcium in your urine, which is a major cause of kidney stone development. Reducing dairy consumption would put less work on kidney's filtration process. However, you may not give up sweetened almond milk.

21. Do not overexpose yourself to contrast dyes in imaging

When you engage in tests in hospitals like radiology procedures like CT scans, angiograms, X-rays, and other radiation imaging, you are exposing yourself to dyes that may cause your kidneys some serious problems. As much as possible, consult your doctor when you engage in these kinds of proceedings.

22. Observe proper intake of antibiotics as prescribed by your physician

Whenever we are prescribed with antibiotics, we tend to cut our intake once we feel that we have been cured of our ailments. Antibiotics, which are usually prescribed for 7 days, should be taken in full until the last day. Otherwise, your kidneys will get damaged. Do not cut it short nor use it beyond the prescribed period.

23. Do your job

Lastly, those are your kidneys. And more than your doctors and anyone else, you are responsible for their health. If you have problems with your kidneys, no matter how mild, consider taking extra precaution and practicing healthier habits.

CONCLUSION

Thank you again for downloading this book!

Our kidneys do their job of filtering our blood off of excess toxins and wastes, producing hormones necessary for our body's growth and development, and regulating our body's water content for 24 hours a day and 7 days a week, with no pay. So, the least and best thing we could do is offer them the kind of care and attention that would keep them in their utmost healthy condition. This is because our kidneys may be prone to different kinds of health problems that may complicate in the long run, most especially if we disregard their need to be taken care of. Diseases like kidney failure, kidney stones development, chronic kidney disease, acute kidney injury, kidney cysts, urinary tract infection, kidney cancer and many other possibilities may affect our kidneys.

Taking care of the kidneys means we should be able to provide them with the proper diet and lifestyle. Proper diet may include opting for healthier, natural, fresh, whole, and organic foods, detoxifying juices, and dismissing processed and highly preserved foods. All these options may not even be cost you much as they can be done naturally and easily in your own kitchens. While lifestyle change may mean letting go of all the unhealthy habits that damage your kidneys like smoking, drinking alcohol excessively, and even resisting the urge to pee when you really need to. Simple changes in diet and lifestyle may even be quite difficult at first but they may be the best keys to achieving kidneys that would function real well to support your body.

In order to avoid all the possibilities of damaging your kidneys in any possible way, it would be best for you to learn about how they actually work and what they really need so you can provide them with the nutrients and support that would allow them to do their jobs well. Our kidneys play a very important role in body. In a large-scale and societal analogy, our kidneys may serve as the police officers in a society that would keep the peace and order in a place by catching criminals and keeping them in jail, of course with due process. Like our kidneys, without this kind of organization and process of keeping things in line, the entire body with be in total chaos and damage.

So, take your decision of taking care of your kidneys by having a healthier diet and lifestyle change now and do not put your kidney's health at risk any longer. This will be the least and best thing that you could do for them.

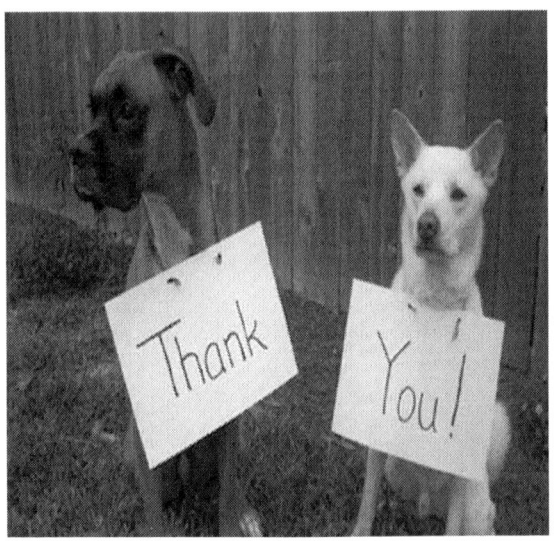

Finally, if you enjoyed this book, then I'd like to ask you for a favor, would you be kind enough to leave a review for this book on Amazon? It'd be greatly appreciated!

Click here to leave a review for this book on Amazon!

Thank you and good luck!

Printed in Great Britain
by Amazon